Diabetic Diet After 50 for Beginners

1500+ Days Low-Carb, Low-Sugar Recipes for Managing Prediabetes and Type 2 Diabetes

Henry Paulsen

Table of Contents

Chapter One

Diabetic Diet

Introduction: Adoption of a New Chapter

Entering your 50s brings a host of new experiences and changes, not the least of which is the way your body manages and reacts to food. For those managing diabetes, these changes may require a new approach to diet and nutrition. This book is designed to be a comprehensive guide for anyone over 50 who want to effectively manage their diabetes through diet. By understanding how your body's needs evolve with age and learning to make informed food choices, you can improve your health, increase your energy levels, and improve your overall quality of life.

Understanding Diabetes After 50

What is Diabetes?

Diabetes is a chronic condition characterized by elevated blood glucose (sugar). This occurs either because the body does not produce enough insulin (a hormone that regulates blood sugar) or because the body's cells do not respond effectively to insulin. There are several types of diabetes:

Type 1 diabetes: An autoimmune condition where the body attacks the insulin-producing cells of the pancreas. This type is usually diagnosed in children and young adults, but can occur at any age.

Type 2 diabetes: The most common type, often developing in adults over 45, but increasingly occurring in the younger population due to lifestyle factors. It involves insulin resistance and often progresses to insulin deficiency.

Prediabetes: A condition where blood sugar levels are higher than normal, but not high enough to be classified as diabetes. It is a critical warning sign and a key opportunity to intervene to prevent the progression of type 2 diabetes.

How Diabetes Affects the Body

Diabetes affects the body in several ways:

Blood sugar levels: Chronically high blood sugar levels can damage blood vessels and nerves.

Insulin resistance: Cells become less responsive to insulin and require more insulin to manage blood sugar levels.

Effect on Organs: Over time, high blood sugar can lead to complications affecting the heart, kidneys, eyes and nerves.

Changes in Your 50s

As you age, your body's physiology changes, which affects how diabetes manifests itself and how it should be treated.

Metabolic shifts

Slower Metabolism: Metabolic rate decreases with age, making weight management more challenging.

Body composition: Loss of muscle mass and increased fat storage can worsen insulin resistance.

Hormonal changes

Menopause: Women experience fluctuations in estrogen and progesterone that affect insulin sensitivity and blood sugar levels.

Andropause: Men may experience a drop in testosterone, which affects muscle mass, fat distribution, and insulin sensitivity.

Increased risk factors

Aging naturally increases the risk of certain conditions that can complicate diabetes management:

Cardiovascular disease: High blood sugar damages blood vessels, increasing the risk of heart disease and stroke.

Neuropathy: Nerve damage can lead to pain, tingling, or loss of sensation, especially in the extremities.

Kidney disease: Diabetes is a leading cause of chronic kidney disease and failure.

Vision problems: Diabetic retinopathy and other vision

problems become more common with age.

Understanding these changes is the first step to adapting your diet and lifestyle to effectively manage diabetes after 50.

Nutritional Needs After 50

As you age, your nutritional needs evolve. Understanding these changes and adjusting your diet can help manage diabetes and maintain overall health. Here's a comprehensive look at essential nutrients and how to incorporate them into your diet.

Macronutrients

Carbohydrates

Carbohydrates are the primary source of energy, but not all carbohydrates are created equal. When treating diabetes, focus on complex carbohydrates, which digest more slowly and have a more subtle effect on blood sugar levels.

Complex carbohydrates: Whole grains, vegetables, legumes, and fruits all contain this compound. These give continuous energy and critical nutrients.

Simple sugars: Avoid or limit foods with added sugars, such as candy, baked goods, and sugary drinks, because they cause rapid spikes in blood sugar.

Tips:

Choose whole grains such as brown rice, quinoa, and whole grain bread.

Include plenty of non-starchy vegetables such as spinach, broccoli and bell peppers.

Proteins

Protein is essential for muscle maintenance, especially since muscle mass tends to decline with age. It also helps manage hunger and keep blood sugar levels stable.

Lean protein: Choose sources such as chicken, turkey, fish, eggs and low-fat dairy products.

Plant-based proteins: Add beans, lentils, tofu, and almonds to your diet.

Tips:

Include a protein source in each meal.

Explore a variety of protein sources to ensure you're getting the full range of amino acids.

Fats

Healthy fats are vital for brain health, hormone production and the absorption of certain vitamins. However, the balance and type of fat is key.

Healthy fats: Look for monounsaturated and polyunsaturated fats in olive oil, avocados, nuts, seeds, and fatty seafood.

Fats to limit: Reduce your intake of saturated fat (found in red meat and full-fat dairy) and avoid trans fat (found in many processed foods).

Tips:

Use olive oil instead of butter for cooking.

Snack on nuts and seeds and add avocado to salads and sandwiches.

Micronutrients

Vitamins and minerals

As you age, your body's ability to absorb certain vitamins and minerals can decrease, so it's important to focus on nutrient-dense foods.

Vitamin D: Supports bone health and immune function. Get it from exposure to sunlight, fortified foods, and oily fish.

Calcium: Essential for bone health. It is found in dairy products, leafy vegetables and fortified plant-based milks.

B vitamins: Required for energy production and neuronal function.

It is found in whole grain products, meat, eggs and dairy products.

Magnesium: Helps with blood sugar control and muscle function. Found in nuts, seeds, whole grains and leafy greens.

Tips:

Consider a vitamin D supplement if you are limited in sun exposure.

Provide a varied diet that covers a wide spectrum of vitamins and minerals.

Fiber

Fiber is crucial for good digestive health and blood sugar control. It helps to slow the absorption of sugar into the bloodstream, thus preventing spikes in blood sugar levels.

Soluble fiber: Found in oats, legumes, apples and citrus fruits. It helps to reduce the level of cholesterol and glucose in the blood.

Insoluble fiber: Found in whole grains, nuts and vegetables. Supports healthy digestion and regular stools.

Tips:

Include high-fiber foods in every meal.

Aim for at least 2530 grams of fiber per day from a variety of sources.

Hydration

Hydration becomes increasingly important as we age, as thirst decreases, and dehydration can worsen problems with blood sugar control.

Water: Aim for at least 8 glasses a day, more if you are physically active.

Other hydration options: Herbal teas, infused water, and limited amounts of coffee and tea.

Tips:

Keep a water bottle with you and sip it throughout the day.

Include hydrating foods such as cucumbers, oranges and strawberries in your diet.

Chapter Two

Building a Diabetes-Friendly Diet

Creating a diabetes-friendly diet involves understanding how different foods affect your blood sugar and making informed choices that support your overall health. It provides practical strategies for planning and preparing meals that are nutritious and delicious.

The Plate Method

The plate method is a simple and effective way to create balanced meals that help manage blood sugar. It involves dividing the plate into specific parts to ensure the right balance of nutrients.

Half the plate: Non-starchy vegetables (e.g. leafy greens, broccoli, peppers, tomatoes)

One-Quarter of the Plate: Lean protein (e.g., chicken, fish, tofu, beans)

One-quarter of a plate: Whole grains or starchy vegetables (e.g., brown rice, quinoa, sweet potatoes)

Optional: A small serving of fruit or dairy on the side

Tips:

Use a 9-inch plate to control portion sizes.

Choose colorful vegetables to ensure a variety of nutrients.

Meal Planning and Preparation

Effective meal planning and preparation can help you maintain a healthy diabetes diet and reduce the temptation to make unhealthy choices.

Weekly Planning

Set aside time: Set aside a specific time each week for meal planning.

Create a meal plan: Plan your breakfast, lunch, dinner and snacks for the week.

Create a shopping list: List the ingredients needed for your planned meals to streamline your grocery shopping.

Tips:

Include a variety of foods to avoid boredom and ensure a range of nutrients.

Make larger portions of certain foods that can be eaten as leftovers.

Smart grocery shopping

Perimeter Store: The outer edges of a grocery store usually contain fresh produce, meat, and dairy products.

Read labels: Pay attention to nutrition labels and ingredient lists to avoid added sugars and unhealthy fats.

Stock up on staples: Keep healthy staples like whole grains, legumes, and frozen vegetables on hand for easy meal prep.

Tips:

Avoid shopping when you're hungry to avoid impulse purchases of unhealthy foods.

Choose fresh seasonal produce for better taste and nutrition.

Healthy Cooking Techniques

Baking, grilling and steaming: These methods preserve nutrients and reduce the need for added fats.

Use herbs and spices: Enhance the taste of your dishes without adding extra salt or sugar.

Tips:

Experiment with various herbs and spices to create novel flavor combinations.

Invest in good quality non-stick cookware to reduce the need for added fats during cooking.

Incorporating Superfoods

Superfoods are nutrient-dense foods that offer numerous health advantages. Including them in your diet can help manage diabetes and improve overall health.

Leafy greens and cruciferous vegetables

Examples: spinach, cabbage, broccoli, cauliflower

Advantages: High content of vitamins, minerals and

antioxidants; low in calories and carbohydrates

Tips:

Add spinach or kale to smoothies for a nutrient boost.

Fry broccoli or cauliflower in a drizzle of olive oil and your favorite spices.

Berries and fruits

Low glycemic options: Blueberries, strawberries, apples

Portion control: Eat fruit in moderation to avoid blood sugar spikes.

Tips:

Top quality Greek yogurt with a handful of berries for a nutritious snack.

Pair apple slices with a spoonful of almond butter for a balanced treat.

Nuts and seeds

Healthy snack: Almonds, chia seeds, flax seeds

Nutrient-Rich Ingredients: Add nuts and seeds to salads, oatmeal or yogurt.

Tips:

For a convenient snack, keep a small container of mixed nuts in your bag.

Sprinkle chia or flax seeds on top of your smoothie or cereal.

Smart Carb Choices

Choosing the right types of carbohydrates can help keep your blood sugar stable and provide sustained energy.

Whole grains

Examples: Quinoa, brown rice, oats

Advantages: High content of fiber, vitamins and minerals; lower glycemic index compared to refined grains

Tips:

Replace white rice with brown rice or quinoa in your meal.

Enjoy a bowl of oatmeal with fresh fruit and nuts for breakfast.

Legumes and beans

Examples: Lentils, chickpeas, black beans

Benefits: High in fiber and protein; they help regulate blood sugar levels

Tips:

Add beans to salads, soups and stews for added protein and fiber.

Make a batch of chickpea hummus for a healthy dip or spread.

Incorporating Protein into Every Meal

Ensuring you get enough protein at every meal helps manage hunger, maintain muscle mass and stabilize blood sugar levels.

Breakfast ideas

Greek yogurt parfait: Greek yogurt with berries and a sprinkle of nuts or seeds

Egg-based dishes: Scrambled eggs with spinach and tomatoes or an omelette with vegetables

Tips:

Make overnight oats with Greek yogurt and chia seeds for a quick protein-rich breakfast.

Keep hard-boiled eggs on hand for a convenient protein snack.

Lunch and dinner

Lean protein sources: Grilled chicken, fish, tofu, beans

Balanced meals: Combine lean protein with vegetables and whole grains.

Tips:

Prepare a large salad with mixed greens, grilled chicken, and a variety of colorful veggies.

Make a stir-fry with tofu, broccoli, peppers and brown rice.

Superfoods for Managing Diabetes

Superfoods are nutrient-dense foods that provide significant health benefits, including helping to manage diabetes by stabilizing blood sugar, reducing inflammation, and improving overall health. Including these foods in your diet can improve your diabetes management plan and support your long-term health goals.

Leafy Greens and Cruciferous Vegetables

Leafy greens and cruciferous vegetables are low in calories and carbohydrates, but high in vitamins, minerals and antioxidants. They are essential for a diabetic-friendly diet due to their nutrient density and low glycemic index.

Spinach and cabbage

Nutritional profile: High in vitamins A, C and K, as well as iron and calcium.

Benefits: Antioxidant, anti-inflammatory and supports bone health.

Tips:

Add fresh spinach or kale to smoothies for a nutrient boost without greatly altering the taste.

Sauté spinach or cabbage with garlic and olive oil as a quick and nutritious side dish.

Broccoli and cauliflower

Nutritional profile: High in vitamins C and K, fiber and folic acid.

Benefits: Contains sulforaphane, which has an anti-inflammatory effect and regulates blood sugar levels.

Tips:

Roast broccoli or cauliflower in a drizzle of olive oil and your favorite herbs for a tasty and healthy side dish.

Include steamed broccoli or cauliflower in salads or stir-fries.

Berries and Fruits

Berries and certain fruits are packed with antioxidants, vitamins, and fiber while also having a low glycemic index, making them an excellent choice for treating diabetes.

Blueberries and strawberries

Nutritional profile: Rich in vitamins C and K, fiber and

antioxidants such as anthocyanins.

Benefits: Help improve insulin sensitivity and reduce blood sugar fluctuations.

Tips:

Add a handful of blueberries or strawberries to Greek yogurt for a nutritious breakfast or snack.

Mix berries into oatmeal or whole grain cereal for added flavor and nutrients.

Apples

Nutritional profile: High in fiber, vitamins C and K and various antioxidants.

Benefits: Fiber slows the absorption of sugar and improves digestion.

Tips:

Slice apples and pair them with a spoonful of almond butter for a balanced snack.

Apple slices make a delicious and crisp accent to salads.

Nuts and Seeds

Nuts and seeds are high in fiber, protein, and healthy fats. They can help manage blood sugar levels and provide sustained energy.

Almonds and walnuts

Nutritional profile: High in monounsaturated fat, protein, fiber and vitamin E.

Benefits: Helps improve heart health and regulate blood sugar.

Tips:

Keep a small container of mixed nuts for a convenient snack.

Add chopped almonds or walnuts to salads, oatmeal or yogurt.

Chia seeds and flax seeds

Nutritional profile: Rich in omega-3 fatty acids, fiber, and protein.

Benefits: Help improve heart health, reduce inflammation and stabilize blood sugar.

Tips:

Sprinkle chia seeds or ground flax seeds on smoothies, yogurt or cereal.

Use chia seeds to make a nutritious pudding by soaking them in almond milk overnight.

Whole Grains and Legumes

Whole grains and legumes are excellent sources of complex carbohydrates, fiber and protein. They have a low glycemic index and give continuous energy.

Quinoa and brown rice

Nutritional profile: High in fiber, protein and various vitamins and minerals.

Benefits: Helps regulate blood sugar levels and supports digestive health.

Tips:

Use quinoa or brown rice as a base for salads, bowls or side dishes.

Cook a batch of quinoa or brown rice at the beginning of the week for easy meal prep.

Lentils and chickpeas

Nutritional profile: High in fiber, protein, iron and folic acid.

Benefits: Helps stabilize blood sugar levels and supports heart health.

Tips:

Add lentils or chickpeas to soups, stews or salads for added protein and fiber.

Make a batch of chickpea hummus for a healthy dip or spread.

Chapter Three

Carbohydrate Management

Carbohydrates are a major source of energy, but managing their intake is essential to controlling diabetes. Understanding the different types of carbohydrates and their effects on blood sugar can help you make informed choices that support your health.

Glycemic Index and Glycemic Load

Glycemic Index (GI)

The glycemic index evaluates foods from 0 to 100 according to how quickly they raise blood sugar. High GI foods are digested quickly and cause a spike in blood sugar, while low GI foods are digested more slowly, resulting in a gradual rise in blood sugar.

Low GI (55 or less): Examples include most fruits and vegetables, legumes, whole grains, and nuts.

Medium GI (5669): Examples include whole grains, sweet potatoes, and brown rice.

High GI (70 or more): Examples include white bread, rice, potatoes, and sugary snacks.

Glycemic Load (GL)

Glycemic load takes into account both the quality (GI) and quantity of carbohydrates in a serving of food, giving a more accurate picture of a food's effect on blood sugar.

Low GL (10 or less): Indicates less impact on blood sugar per serving.

Medium GL (1119): Moderate impact.

High GL (20 or more): High impact.

Tips:

Aim for low to medium GI foods to keep your blood sugar stable.

Use GL as a tool to help control portions, even when eating high GI foods.

Smart Carb Choices

Choosing the right types of carbohydrates is essential to managing diabetes. Emphasize whole, unprocessed foods that provide fiber, vitamins and minerals.

Whole grains

Whole grains are minimally processed and contain all parts of the grain kernel, making them higher in fiber and nutrients than refined grains.

Examples: Quinoa, brown rice, whole wheat, barley, oats.

Benefits: High in fiber, which helps slow down digestion and the release of glucose into the bloodstream.

Tips:

Replace white rice with brown rice or quinoa.

Choose whole grain breads, pastas and cereals over refined versions.

Legumes and beans

Legumes and beans are excellent sources of complex carbohydrates, fiber and protein.

They have a low GI and can assist
to regulate blood sugar levels.

Examples: Lentils, chickpeas,
black beans, kidney beans.

Benefits: High in fiber and protein
to help regulate blood sugar and
provide a feeling of fullness.

Tips:

Add beans to soups, salads and
stews for added nutrition.

Make a batch of lentils or
chickpeas for easy meal additions
throughout the week.

Portion and Frequency Management

Portion control and meal timing are key strategies for managing carbohydrate intake and blood sugar levels.

Portion control

Visual cues: Use your hand or common objects to estimate portion sizes. For example, one serving of rice or pasta should be about the size of a tennis ball.

The Plate Method: Fill half your plate with non-starchy vegetables, one-quarter with lean protein, and one-quarter with whole grains or starchy vegetables.

Tips:

First, measure portions to better understand the appropriate portion size.

To prevent overeating, avoid eating directly from huge packages.

Meal timing

Regular meals: Eating at a consistent time every day helps keep blood sugar levels stable.

Balanced meals: Include a mix of carbohydrates, protein and

healthy fats at each meal to slow down the absorption of sugar.

Tips:

Don't skip meals as this can lead to overeating later and cause blood spikes.

Include snacks between meals if you have long gaps between them to prevent blood sugar from dropping.

Smart substitutions

Smart substitutions can help reduce the glycemic impact of your meals.

Low glycemic alternatives

Zucchini Noodles (Zoodles): Use instead of pasta.

Cauliflower rice: Use instead of white or brown rice.

Sweet potatoes: Use in place of regular potatoes for a lower GI option.

Tips:

Experiment with vegetable-based alternatives to lower your carb intake.

Use these substitutes in your favorite recipes to maintain flavor and texture while managing carbs.

Monitoring and Adjusting

Regularly monitoring and adjusting your diet based on your blood sugar levels can help you find the right balance of carbohydrates.

Blood sugar monitoring

Track your levels: Keep a record of your pre-meal and post-meal blood sugar readings.

Identify patterns: Notice how different foods and portions affect your blood sugar.

Tips:

Consult your healthcare practitioner to discover your ideal blood sugar range.

Use your blood sugar data to make informed dietary adjustments.

Protein Power

Protein plays a vital role in managing diabetes, especially as you age. It helps maintain muscle mass, boosts metabolism and provides a feeling of fullness that can help regulate appetite and blood sugar levels. This will explore the importance of protein, how much you need and the best sources to include in your diet.

The Importance of Protein

Protein is essential for a number of bodily functions, including:

Muscle maintenance: Helps preserve muscle mass, which naturally decreases with age.

Blood sugar control: It slows down the absorption of carbohydrates and prevents a rapid rise in blood sugar.

Satiety: Promotes a feeling of fullness, which can help with weight management and prevent overeating.

Metabolism: Supports a healthy metabolism, helps with weight control and energy balance.

How much protein do you need?

Your protein requirements are determined by a number of factors, including your age, degree of activity, and overall health. As a general guideline, focus on:

Daily intake: About 0.8 grams of protein per kilogram of body weight (0.36 grams per pound). For someone who weighs 70 kg (154 pounds), that means about 56 grams of protein per day.

Increased needs: Older adults may benefit from higher protein intake to prevent muscle loss.

Aim for 1.0 to 1.2 grams per kilogram of body weight (0.45 to 0.54 grams per pound).

Tips:

Spread your protein intake evenly throughout the day to promote muscle synthesis and blood sugar control.

Include protein in each meal and snack.

Best Sources of Protein

Including a variety of protein sources in your diet will ensure you get a range of essential amino acids and other nutrients.

Animal Proteins

Animal proteins are complete proteins, which mean they include all of the required amino acids.

Lean meat

Examples: Chicken, turkey, lean cuts of beef and pork.

Advantages: High in protein, low in saturated fat when choosing lean cuts.

Tips:

Grill, bake or broil meat instead of frying it to reduce the amount of added fat.

Remove the skin from the poultry to reduce the fat content.

Fish and seafood

Examples: salmon, tuna, mackerel, shrimp.

Benefits: Rich in omega-3 fatty acids, which support heart health and reduce inflammation.

Tips:

Aim for at least two servings of oily fish per week.

Try grilling or baking fish with herbs and lemon for added flavor.

Eggs and milk

Examples: Eggs, Greek yogurt, cottage cheese, low-fat milk.

Benefits: Eggs are versatile and rich in nutrients; dairy products provide calcium and vitamin D.

Tips:

Enjoy boiled eggs as a snack or add eggs to salads and sandwiches.

Choose Greek yogurt for higher protein and less added sugars.

Plant-Based Proteins

Plant-based proteins are often lower in calories and saturated fat and provide fiber and other beneficial nutrients.

Legumes and beans

Examples: Lentils, chickpeas, black beans, soybeans.

Benefits: High in protein, fiber and essential nutrients like iron and folate.

Tips:

Use beans as a base for salads, soups and stews.

Make chickpea hummus for a healthy dip or spread.

Nuts and seeds

Examples: Almonds, walnuts, chia seeds, flax seeds, hemp seeds.

Benefits: Provide healthy fats, protein and fiber.

Tips:

Add nuts and seeds to oatmeal, yogurt or salads for added crunch and nutrition.

Make chia seed pudding by soaking chia seeds overnight in almond milk.

Tofu and Tempeh

Examples: Firm tofu, tempeh.

Benefits: Soy-based proteins that is versatile and nutrient-dense.

Tips:

Marinate and grill tofu or tempeh for a tasty source of protein.

Add chopped tofu to stir-fries, soups or salads.

Incorporating Protein into Your Diet

Ensuring you get enough protein at every meal can help manage diabetes and promote overall health.

Breakfast ideas

Greek yogurt parfait: Greek yogurt with berries and a sprinkle of nuts or seeds.

Egg-based dishes: Scrambled eggs with spinach and tomatoes or an omelette with vegetables.

Smoothies: Mix protein powder, Greek yogurt, or silken tofu with fruits and vegetables.

Lunch and dinner

Lean protein sources: Grilled chicken, fish, tofu, beans.

Balanced meals: Combine lean protein with vegetables and whole grains.

Salads: Add a protein source like grilled chicken, tofu, or beans to your salads.

Snacks

Hard Boiled Eggs: Keep a batch of hard boiled eggs for a quick and easy snack.

Nuts and seeds: A handful of almonds, walnuts, or a mix of nuts.

Milk: Cottage cheese or Greek yogurt with a handful of berries.

Chapter Four

Fats and Diabetes

Fats are an essential part of a balanced diet and play a vital role in overall health and diabetes management. Understanding the different types of fats and how to incorporate healthy fats into your diet can help maintain blood sugar levels, promote heart health, and promote overall well-being.

The Role of Fats in the Body

Fats perform several important functions in the body:

Energy Source: Fats supply a concentrated source of energy.

Absorption of nutrients: Fats help absorb fat-soluble vitamins (A, D, E, and K).

Cell function: Fats are vital to the structure and function of cell membranes.

Hormone production: Fats are involved in the production of hormones that regulate various body functions.

Types of Fats

Not all fats are created equal. Understanding the different types of fats and their effects on health is essential to managing diabetes.

Healthy fats

Monounsaturated fats

Sources: Olive oil, avocado, nuts (almonds, cashews, peanuts), seeds (pumpkin, sesame).

Benefits: Help improve blood cholesterol levels, reduce inflammation and provide antioxidants.

Tips:

Use olive oil for cooking and salad dressings.

Snack on a small handful of nuts or add them to salads and yogurts.

Polyunsaturated fats

Sources: Fatty fish (salmon, mackerel, sardines), flax seeds, chia seeds, walnuts, sunflower seeds and oils (soybean, corn, safflower).

Benefits: Include essential omega3 and omega6 fatty acids that support heart health, reduce inflammation and improve insulin sensitivity.

Tips:

Aim for at least two servings of oily fish per week.

Sprinkle flax seeds or chia seeds on oatmeal, yogurt or smoothies.

Fats to Limit

Saturated fats

Sources: Red meat, full-fat dairy products (butter, cheese, cream), coconut oil, palm oil.

Effects: May raise LDL (bad) cholesterol and increase the risk of heart disease.

Tips:

Select lean slices of meat and trim away any visible fat.

Opt for low-fat or fat-free dairy products.

Trans fats

Sources: Partially hydrogenated oils found in some processed and fried foods, baked goods and margarine.

Effects: Increase LDL cholesterol and decrease HDL (good) cholesterol, increasing the risk of heart disease and inflammation.

Tips:

Avoid foods with "partially hydrogenated oils" on the ingredients list.

Instead of frying items, go for baked or grilled options.

Include Healthy Fats in Your Diet

Including healthy fats in your diet can help manage blood sugar levels and improve overall health.

Cooking with healthy fats

Olive oil: Use for sautéing vegetables, dressing salads and marinating meat.

Avocado Oil: Suitable for high temperature cooking such as frying and grilling.

Tips:

Replace butter or margarine with olive oil in recipes.

Experiment with different oils to find your favorite flavors.

Adding healthy fats to meals

Breakfast: Add avocado slices to toast or eggs.

Lunch: Include nuts or seeds in salads and grain bowls.

Dinner: Use fatty fish as your main protein source and cook with healthy oils.

Tips:

Make simple vinaigrette with olive oil, vinegar and herbs for salads.

Add a spoonful of flax seeds or chia seeds to yogurt or oatmeal.

Healthy snacks

Nut Butter: Spread almond or peanut butter on apple slices or whole grain crackers.

Trail Mix: Make a trail mix with nuts, seeds and a small amount of dried fruit.

Tips:

To avoid eating too many calories, keep your portion sizes in check.

Choose natural nut butters that do not contain added sweeteners or hydrogenated oils.

Balancing Fat Intake with Other Nutrients

While healthy fats are beneficial, balancing them with carbohydrates and protein is essential for optimal diabetes management.

Diet: Aim for balanced meals that include a source of healthy fats, lean protein and fiber-rich carbohydrates.

Snacks: Combine healthy fats with protein and fiber for satisfying snacks that stabilize blood sugar.

Tips:

Pair avocado with a lean protein like chicken or tofu for a balanced meal.

Snack on a small handful of nuts with a piece of fruit to keep you energized.

The Role of Fiber

Fiber is a key component of a diabetes-friendly diet and offers a number of health benefits that help manage blood sugar, support digestion and promote overall well-being. This will explore the importance of fibre, its types and how to incorporate fiber rich foods into your diet.

Understanding fiber

Fiber is a form of carbohydrate that the body can't digest. It passes through the digestive system relatively intact, providing bulk and assisting with various bodily functions.

Types of Fibers

Soluble fiber

Sources: Oats, barley, nuts, seeds, beans, lentils, peas and some fruits and vegetables.

Benefits: Soluble fiber dissolves in water to form a gel-like substance that helps lower cholesterol and blood glucose levels. It can slow down the absorption of sugar, helping to regulate blood sugar levels.

Insoluble fiber

Sources: Whole grains, wheat bran, vegetables and whole fruits.

Benefits: Insoluble fiber adds bulk to the stool and helps food pass through the stomach and intestines more quickly. It encourages regular bowel motions and prevents constipation.

Health Benefits of Fiber for Diabetes

Including fiber in your diet offers several benefits, especially for those with diabetes:

Blood sugar control

Slow absorption: Fiber slows the absorption of sugar and prevents a rapid rise in blood sugar.

Improved insulin sensitivity: High-fiber diets can improve insulin sensitivity and help the body use insulin more efficiently.

Weight management

Satiety: Fiber promotes feelings of fullness, which can help control appetite and reduce overall calorie intake.

Reduced calorie density: Foods high in fiber are usually lower in calories, making them beneficial for weight management.

Heart health

Lowering Cholesterol: Soluble fiber can help lower LDL (bad) cholesterol and reduce the risk of heart disease.

Blood pressure: High-fiber diets are associated with lower blood pressure levels.

Digestive health

Regularity: Insoluble fiber helps prevent constipation and promotes regular bowel movements.

Gut health: Fiber acts as a prebiotic, nourishing beneficial gut bacteria and supporting a healthy microbiome.

How much fiber do you need?

The necessary daily fiber intake varies depending on age and gender, but a common guideline is:

Men (50 and older): About 30 grams of fiber each day.

Women (50 and older): About 21 grams of fiber per day.

Tips:

Gradually increase your fiber intake to avoid digestive problems.

Drink plenty of water to assist fiber pass through your digestive tract.

Including Fiber-Rich Foods in Your Diet

Whole grains

Whole grains include high levels of soluble and insoluble fiber.

Examples: oats, barley, quinoa, brown rice, whole wheat, bulgur.

Benefits: Whole grains provide essential nutrients, including B vitamins, iron and magnesium.

Tips:

Start your day with a bowl of oatmeal with berries and nuts.

Choose whole grain breads, pastas and cereals over refined versions.

Fruits and vegetables

Fruits and vegetables are rich in fiber, vitamins and minerals.

Examples: apples, pears, berries, oranges, carrots, broccoli, spinach, sweet potatoes.

Benefits: They provide a variety of nutrients and antioxidants that support overall health.

Tips:

If possible, keep the skins on fruits and vegetables, as they contain significant amounts of fiber.

Snack on raw vegetables and hummus, or a piece of fruit.

Legumes

Legumes are high in both soluble and insoluble fiber, making them an excellent choice for a high-fiber diet.

Examples: Beans, lentils, chickpeas, peas.

Benefits: They also provide protein, making them a great plant-based source of protein.

Tips:

Add beans to soups, stews and salads.

Make a lentil-based dish for a high-fiber, high-protein meal.

Nuts and seeds

Nuts and seeds offer a good amount of fiber along with healthy fats and protein.

Examples: Almonds, chia seeds, flax seeds, sunflower seeds.

Benefits: They are nutritious and can keep you full between meals.

Tips:

Sprinkle the seeds on yogurt, oatmeal, or salads.

Enjoy a handful of nuts or add them to baked goods.

Practical Tips for Increasing Fiber Intake

Increase gradually: Increase your fiber intake slowly to allow your digestive system to adjust.

Hydration: Drink plenty of water to help fiber move through your digestive system.

Balanced diet: Combine high-fiber foods with protein and healthy fats for balanced meals.

Tips:

Add fiber-rich foods to your meals and snacks throughout the day.

Experiment with new recipes that include different sources of fiber.

Chapter Five

Hydration and Diabetes

Proper hydration is essential for everyone, but it is especially important for individuals struggling with diabetes. Staying well hydrated helps regulate blood sugar, supports kidney function and contributes to overall well-being. It will explore the role of hydration in the management of diabetes and provide practical tips for maintaining adequate hydration.

The Importance of Hydration

Hydration plays several essential roles in the body:

Blood sugar regulation: Water helps dilute glucose in the bloodstream, which can help control blood sugar.

Kidney function: Proper hydration supports kidney function, which is essential for filtering waste products, including excess glucose.

Digestion: Water aids digestion and helps prevent constipation.

Circulation: Adequate hydration supports blood circulation and nutrient transport.

Temperature regulation: Water helps regulate body temperature through sweating and breathing.

Hydration and Blood Sugar Level

Dehydration can have a significant impact on blood sugar levels and overall diabetes management:

Elevated blood sugar: Dehydration can lead to higher blood sugar levels because the concentration of glucose in the blood increases.

Decreased insulin sensitivity: Dehydration can decrease insulin sensitivity, making it harder for the body to use insulin effectively.

Tips:

Monitor your blood sugar regularly, especially during periods of hot weather or increased physical activity, to ensure you stay hydrated.

Drink water throughout the day to maintain consistent hydration and support blood sugar regulation.

How much water do you need?

The amount of water you need can vary depending on factors such as age, gender, activity level and climate. However, general guidelines include:

Men: About 3.7 liters (125 ounces) of total water per day, including all drinks and food.

Women: About 2.7 liters (91 ounces) of total water per day, including all beverages and food.

Tips:

Listen to your body and drink water as soon as you feel thirsty.

Increase water intake during hot weather, physical activity, or illness to compensate for increased water loss.

Best Hydration Practices for Diabetes

Drink a Lot of Water

Water is the best choice for staying hydrated. It is calorie-free, readily available, and essential for many bodily functions.

Tips:

Carry a reusable water bottle with you throughout the day to encourage consistent water consumption.

Set a reminder on your phone or use a water tracking app to help you meet your hydration goals.

Limit sugary drinks

Sugary drinks such as sodas, fruit juices and sugary drinks can cause rapid spikes in blood sugar and contribute to dehydration.

Tips:

Replace sugary drinks with water, herbal teas or infused water for a healthier alternative.

If you like the taste of fruit juices, dilute them with water to reduce the sugar content.

Be careful with caffeinated and alcoholic beverages

Caffeinated and alcoholic beverages can have diuretic properties, resulting in increased urine output and possible dehydration.

Tips:

Balance out caffeinated drinks like coffee and tea with plenty of water to stay hydrated.

Drink alcohol in moderation and alternate it with water to maintain hydration levels.

Eat hydrating foods

Many fruits and vegetables are high in water content and can contribute to your overall hydration.

Examples: cucumbers, watermelon, strawberries, oranges, lettuce, celery and tomatoes.

Benefits: These foods provide hydration and essential vitamins, minerals and fiber.

Tips:

Include hydrating fruits and vegetables in your meals and snacks.

Make salads with vegetables high in water content for a refreshing and hydrating meal.

Monitor your hydration status

Watch for signs of dehydration and adjust your water intake as needed.

Symptoms of dehydration: Dark yellow urine, dry mouth, fatigue, dizziness and headaches.

Urine Color: A light, pale yellow color usually indicates adequate hydration.

Tips:

Check the color of your urine regularly as a simple way to gauge your hydration status.

Increase your water intake if you notice signs of dehydration.

Special consideration for older adults

As you age, your thirst may decrease, making it even more

important to consciously drink enough water.

Tips:

Schedule regular water breaks throughout the day to ensure consistent hydration.

Keep a water bottle close at hand as a reminder to drink.

Special Considerations and Tips

Managing diabetes requires individualized care and attention to the various factors that can affect your health and well-being. This will cover special considerations and practical tips to improve your diabetes management plan and promote a healthy lifestyle.

1. Regular monitoring

Monitoring your blood sugar regularly is essential to understanding how food, physical activity, medications and other factors affect your body. Work with your healthcare team to establish target ranges and determine the frequency of monitoring that is right for you.

Tips:

Keep a log of your blood sugar readings and share them with your healthcare provider during visits.

Use a blood glucose meter or continuous glucose monitor (CGM) to track trends and make informed decisions about diabetes management.

2. Medication adherence

Taking the medications prescribed by your healthcare provider is essential for effective diabetes management. This includes insulin injections, oral medications, and other treatments prescribed to control blood sugar.

Tips:

Set a reminder on your phone or use a pill organizer to make sure you take your medication on time.

Communicate openly with your healthcare team about any problems or concerns you have about your medications.

3. Coping with stress

Stress has been shown to have an impact on blood sugar levels and general health. Finding healthy ways to manage stress is essential to managing diabetes.

Tips:

Deep breathing, meditation, and yoga are all effective relaxation strategies.

Engage in hobbies or activities you enjoy to reduce stress and promote relaxation.

4. Quality of sleep

Sufficient quality sleep is important for managing diabetes. Poor sleep can affect blood sugar levels, appetite and overall health.

Tips:

Maintain a consistent sleep schedule by going to bed and getting up at the same time each day.

Create a relaxing bedtime routine and avoid stimulating activities, caffeine and screens before bed.

5. Foot care

People with diabetes are at risk for foot problems due to nerve damage and reduced blood flow to the feet. Proper Foot care is vital for avoiding issues.

Tips:

Check your feet daily for cuts, sores, or signs of infection.

Keep your feet clean and moisturized, and wear shoes that fit well and are comfortable.

6. Dental and oral health

Diabetes can increase the risk of gum disease and other oral health problems. Good dental hygiene is important for overall health.

Tips:

Brush your teeth at least twice a day, and floss everyday.
Schedule frequent dental exams and cleanings with your dentist.

7. Social support

Managing diabetes can be challenging, but having a strong support system can make a big difference. Surround yourself with supportive friends, family members, or join a diabetes support group.

Tips:

Share your experiences and challenges with people who understand your situation.

Attend diabetes classes or workshops to learn from experts and connect with others.

8. Travel

Traveling with diabetes requires planning and preparation to ensure you have everything you need to manage your condition away from home.

Tips:

Pack extra supplies, including medications, insulin, testing supplies, and snacks.

Carry a letter from your healthcare provider explaining your condition and any necessary medical supplies.

9. Emergency Preparedness

Prepare for emergencies by having a diabetes emergency kit and knowing what to do in case of high or low blood sugar.

Tips:

Keep emergency contact information and medical information readily available.

Carry glucose tablets or fast-acting carbohydrates to treat low blood sugar.

10. Regular health care visits

Schedule regular checkups with your healthcare provider to monitor your diabetes management, review your treatment plan, and address any concerns or questions you may have.

Tips:

Prepare a list of questions or topics to discuss during the meetings.

Be proactive in managing your health by following your provider's recommendations and making adjustments as needed.

Recipes and Meal Plans

Here are some diabetes-friendly recipes and meal planning tips to help you maintain a balanced diet and manage your blood sugar effectively.

Breakfast Recipes

Greek Yogurt Parfait

Ingredients:

1/2 cup Greek yogurt (plain, unsweetened)

1/4 cup berries (such as strawberries, blueberries, or raspberries)

1 tablespoon chopped nuts (almonds, walnuts)

1 teaspoon honey or maple syrup
(optional)

Instruction:

1. Layer Greek yogurt, berries
and chopped nuts in a serving
glass or bowl.

2. Drizzle with honey or maple
syrup as desired.

3. Enjoy immediately or
refrigerate for later.

Veggie Omelette

Ingredients:

2 eggs

1/4 cup chopped bell pepper (red,
green, yellow)

1/4 cup chopped tomatoes

1 tablespoon diced onion

Salt and pepper to taste

Cooking spray or olive oil for
cooking

Instruction:

1. In a mixing bowl, whisk the
eggs until well blended. Season
with salt and pepper.

2. Heat a nonstick skillet over
medium heat and coat with
cooking spray or olive oil.

3. Add the chopped vegetables to
the pan and cook until tender,
about 34 minutes.

4. Pour the beaten eggs over the vegetables and cook until the eggs are set, about 23 minutes.

5. Fold the omelet in half and transfer to a plate. Serve hot.

Recipes for Lunch

Grilled Chicken Salad

Ingredients:

1 boneless skinless chicken breast

Mixed vegetable salad (lettuce, spinach)

1/2 cup cherry tomatoes, halved

1/4 cucumber, sliced

1/4 avocado, sliced

Balsamic vinaigrette dressing
(olive oil, balsamic vinegar, Dijon
mustard, salt, pepper)

Instruction:

1. Preheat the grill or grill pan to
medium-high temperature.

2. Salt and pepper the chicken
breast. Grill for 57 minutes on
each side until cooked through.

3. Allow the chicken to rest for a
few minutes before slicing.

4. Place green salad, cherry
tomatoes, cucumber and avocado
in a large bowl.

5. Top with sliced grilled chicken and drizzle with balsamic vinaigrette dressing.

Quinoa and Black Bean Stuffed Bell Peppers

Ingredients:

2 bell peppers (of any color), halved and seeded

1/2 cup quinoa, cooked

1/2 cup black beans, drained and rinsed

1/4 cup corn kernels (fresh or frozen)

1/4 cup chopped tomatoes

1/4 teaspoon cumin

Salt and pepper to taste

Instruction:

1. Preheat oven to 375°F (190°C).

2. In a bowl, combine the cooked quinoa, black beans, corn kernels, diced tomatoes, cumin, salt and pepper.

3. Fill each pepper halfway with the quinoa mixture.

4. Place the stuffed peppers on a baking sheet and bake for 2025 minutes until the peppers are soft.

5. Serve warm as a nutritious lunch.

Recipes for Dinner

Baked Salmon with Asparagus

Ingredients:

2 salmon fillets

1 bunch asparagus, chopped

1 tablespoon of olive oil

1 lemon, cut into slices

Salt and pepper to taste

Instruction:

1. Preheat oven to 400°F (200°C).

2. Place the salmon fillets and asparagus on a baking sheet lined with baking paper.

3. Drizzle the salmon and asparagus with olive oil. Season with salt and pepper.

4. Place the lemon slices on top of the salmon.

5. Bake for 1520 minutes until the salmon is cooked and the asparagus is tender.

6. Serve hot alongside brown rice or quinoa.

Stir-Fried Tofu with Vegetables

Ingredients:

1 firm block of tofu, drained and diced

1 cup mixed vegetables (pepper, broccoli, peas)

2 tablespoons low-sodium soy sauce

1 tablespoon hoisin sauce

1 teaspoon of sesame oil

1 clove of garlic, chopped

1/2 teaspoon grated ginger

Cooking spray or olive oil for cooking

Instruction:

1. Heat a non-stick pan or wok over medium-high heat. Coat with cooking spray or olive oil.

2. Add the sliced tofu to the pan and fry until golden brown on all sides, about 57 minutes. Remove from pan and set aside.

3. Add chopped garlic and grated ginger to the same pan. Fry for 1 minute until fragrant.

4. Add the mixed vegetables to the pan and stir for 34 minutes until golden.

5. Return the tofu to the pan. Add low sodium soy sauce, hoisin sauce and sesame oil. Stir for another 23 minutes until heated through.

6. Serve hot with brown rice or whole wheat noodles.

Tips for Meal Planning

Balance your plate: Include a variety of foods from different food groups at each meal; vegetables, lean protein, whole grains, and healthy fats.

Portion control: Pay attention to portion sizes to avoid overeating and keep your blood sugar stable.

Snack Smart: Choose healthy snacks like fruit, nuts, yogurt or vegetables with hummus to stave off hunger between meals.

Plan Ahead: Prepare meals and snacks ahead of time so you have nutritious options available and reduce the temptation to make unhealthy choices.

Stay hydrated: Drink water throughout the day to stay hydrated and promote overall health.

By incorporating these recipes and meal planning tips into your routine, you can enjoy delicious and satisfying meals while effectively managing your diabetes. Adjust the recipes to suit your preferences and consult with your healthcare provider or registered dietitian for individualized guidance based on your individual needs.

Conclusion

Embracing a diabetic diet after 50 doesn't mean giving up the joy of eating; it's about making smart, informed decisions that support your health and well-being. By incorporating the principles and tips outlined in this book, you can effectively manage your diabetes and enjoy a vibrant and active life well into your later years.